Bread Machine Cookbook for your Holiday

50 delicious bread recipes for your holiday, affordable and easy to prepare

Raul Wyatt

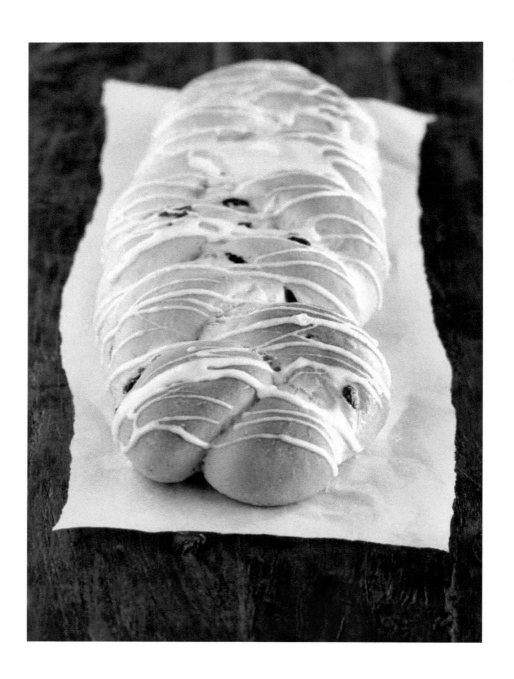

COPYRIGHT

Table of Contents

Seeded Pumpkin Baguette

Preparation Time: 10 min. + 1h. 30 min.

1-Pound Loaf

Ingredients:

For the bread:

· 1½ cups pumpkin puree

· 2 teaspoons instant yeast

· 2 teaspoons honey

· ½ cup lukewarm water

· 2 teaspoons vegetable oil

· 3½ cups all-purpose flour

· ½ cup sunflower seeds

· 2 teaspoons sesame seeds

· 1 tablespoon flax seeds

· 2 teaspoons salt

For the topping:

· 1 egg lightly beaten

· ¼ cup pepitas pumpkin seeds

· 1 tablespoon poppy seeds

· 2 tablespoons sunflower seeds

Directions:

1. In the stand mixer bowl (with paddle attachment) add the pumpkin puree, honey, yeast, water, oil, and 1 cup of flour. Mix well to combine at a low speed. Add the seeds and salt. Then, set the kneading hook. Slowly add in 2 cups of flour, kneading until fully incorporated. Add more flour if you still haven't got a moist and smooth dough. Transfer the dough to a well-oiled bowl, cover with plastic wrap and leave for 60-90 minutes to rise.

2.Place dough onto a floured surface and carefully deflate. Then, divide the dough evenly into 6 pieces and form each one into a 1½" wide and 1½" long log. Transfer them onto a large greased baking sheet. Cover using a kitchen towel and leave for 30-45 minutes.

3.Preheat the oven to 400° F.

4.Brush your bread with beaten egg and sprinkle with sunflower seeds, pepitas, and poppy seeds.

5.Bake for 25 minutes or longer to get a deeper crust.

6.Take the baguettes out of the oven and allow them to completely cool on a cooling rack.

Nutrition:

· Calories: 229

· Carbohydrates:15g

· Fat:17 g

Wheat Shaft Baguette

Preparation Time: 1 min. + 2 h.

3-Pound Loaf

Ingredients:

· 1½ tablespoons granulated yeast

· 1½ tablespoons kosher salt

· 3 cups lukewarm water

· 6½ cups bread flour, plus more for the work surface and shaping

Directions:

1.Mix the yeast, water, and salt in a large bowl. Add the flour and mix with a stand mixer (paddle attachment). Cover using a kitchen towel and leave for 2 hours to double in size.

2.Next, flour the surface of the dough and cut off a ½-pound portion. Flour a piece of dough and form a ball: stretch its surface around the bottom while rotating the dough a quarter-turn as you go. Leave the dough for 5 minutes.

3.Form a rectangle of sorts from the ball. Next, using the palms of your hands, carefully roll it into a 1¼" baguette. Save the rest of the unused dough in the fridge. Turn over the baking sheet and line it with parchment paper. Transfer your dough onto it and leave for 40 minutes to rise.

4.Put another baking sheet in the middle of the oven and roasting pan in the bottom of the oven. Preheat it to 450° F.

5.Dust your dough with flour. Cover the blades of your kitchen scissors with oil and cut into the dough crosswise near the top of the baguette shape, at an angle of 25° to the dough and stopping a quarter inch from its bottom. Fold every cut part over to the side while alternating sides with every cut. Repeat to cut the entire pound.

6.Gently transfer the pound onto the baking sheet and pour 1 cup of hot water into the pan. Close the oven and bake for 25-30 minutes or longer for a deeper color.

7.Remove the baguette from the oven and let it cool completely before serving.

Nutrition:

· Calories: 234

· Carbohydrates: 46 g

· Fat: 1 g

· Protein: 1½ g

· Sodium: 350 mg

Classic Ciabatta

Preparation Time: 10 minutes + 1½ hours

2-Pound Loaf

Ingredients:

· 3½ cups unbleached, unbromated white bread flour

· 1½ teaspoons fine sea salt

· 1 teaspoon instant dry yeast

· 1½ cups warm water 65°F, + 2 teaspoons water

· 1 tablespoon extra-virgin olive oil

Directions:

1.Mix the yeast, flour, and salt in a large bowl, add half of the water into the mixer bowl (using the dough hook). Add all of the dry ingredients and mix at a low speed. Quickly pour in enough of the rest of the water in a slow stream to get a soft and moist dough. Stop mixing and scrape down the hook and the sides of the bowl with a spatula. Mix for 5 more minutes when you've added all the water.

2.Next, mix for 4 minutes on a medium-low speed while adding 1 tsp of olive oil. Mix for 1 more minute until the oil has been fully incorporated. The dough should be smooth and soft with a moist surface. Cover and leave for 3 hours, with a fold after each hour.

3.Oil a large bowl with extra olive oil and put your dough into it. Using your hands, pull one edge, fold it to the center, and lightly press down. Turn the bowl and repeat for the rest of the edges to form a ball. Turn the ball in the bowl to coat it with oil. Leave the dough for 3 hours, folding each hour.

4.Flour a work surface well. Dust the top of the dough and place it onto the work surface. Lightly dust all the sides of the dough and let it rest for 30 seconds.

5.Form a large rectangle from the dough. Put it in a floured couche and cover. Leave for 45-60 minutes, but keep an eye on the dough and determine whether it is ready to be baked. With your fingertip, make dents in the center of the dough. If it slowly and evenly disappears, you can bake it.

6.Put a baking stone on the bottom rack and preheat the oven to 450° F.

7.Line a bread peel with parchment paper. Transfer the bread to the peel, top side up. Place the dough on the parchment paper onto the middle of the stone. Cover it with a large stainless-steel bowl and close the oven. Bake for 5minutes then remove the bowl. Bake for 15 more minutes to get a golden ciabatta.

8.Take out of the oven and put the ciabatta on a cooling rack. Let it cool completely before slicing.

Nutrition:

· Calories: 169

· Carbohydrates: 25 g

· Fat:1 g

No-Knead Ciabatta

Preparation Time: 10 minutes + 11 ½ h.

2 -Pound Loaf

Ingredients:

· 4 cups unbleached all-purpose flour

· 1½ teaspoons kosher salt

· ¼ teaspoon active dry yeast

· 2 cups water

· 1 tablespoon olive oil

· 2 tablespoons cornmeal

Directions:

1.Mix the yeast, flour, and salt in a large bowl. Add the water and mix well, using a rubber spatula. Cover with foil and leave for 11 ½ hours at room temperature.

2.Next, oil a rimmed baking sheet with a brush, dust with cornmeal and set aside.

3.Wipe the work surface with water and line it with a piece of plastic wrap. Flour it to prevent the dough from sticking.

4.Place your dough onto the floured plastic wrap. Press and form a long flat pound from the dough. Next, flip your dough over on

14

the prepared sheet pan using the plastic wrap. Lightly dust the top of the ciabatta with flour and cover with a kitchen towel for 2 hours.

5.Preheat the oven to 425° F. Put the rack in the lower third position. When it's preheated, transfer the sheet pan into the oven. Bake for 25-30 minutes or more until you get a beautiful deep golden crust.

6.Remove from the oven and let the ciabatta to cool completely before slicing on a cooling

7.rack.

Nutrition:

· Calories: 171

· Carbohydrates:8 g

· Fat:1 g

· Protein:2 g

· Sodium: 360 mg

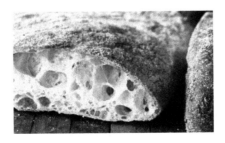

Quick Ciabatta

Preparation Time: 30 minutes + 3 hours.

2-Pound Loaf

Ingredients:

· 4 cups all-purpose flour

· 2¼ teaspoons active dry yeast

· 2¼ cups warm water

· 1 teaspoon salt

· ¼ teaspoon sugar

Directions:

1.Mix the yeast, sugar, and water in a mixing bowl and set aside for 5 minutes. Add the flour and salt and mix in a stand mixer with a paddle. You should get almost a pancake batter, only thicker.

2.Let it stand for 15 minutes. Then mix it at a medium-high speed for 6 minutes. Next, switch the paddle to the dough hook and mix for 6 more minutes to make the dough smooth and not sticking to the bowl.

3.Grease another bowl with oil and put the dough inside. Cover using a kitchen towel and leave for 2 hours in a warm place to triple in size. While it's rising, line a baking sheet with parchment paper and then dust it with flour.

4.Place your dough on the center of the baking sheet and flour the top. Divide the dough evenly into two pieces with a bench scraper. Also, use it and wet hand to shape the dough-tuck every irregular part underneath to get two flat logs. The logs should be about 6" apart. Remember that wet dough doesn't hold a definite shape, so you don't need to shape it perfectly.

5.Dust the tops with flour and cover using a kitchen towel for 1 hour to rise.

6.Preheat your oven to 500°F, keeping the baking stone inside for 30 minutes. Place a pan on the bottom rack.

7.Place the loaves on the baking stone by sliding the parchment off the sheet and pour hot water into the pan, close the oven. Bake for 25 minutes or until the bread has a golden-brown color.

8.Remove from the oven and cool for 40 minutes before slicing.

Nutrition:

· Calories: 172

· Carbohydrates: 28 g

· Fat: 1 g

· Protein: 2 g

· Sodium: 240 mg

Whole-Wheat Ciabatta

Preparation Time: 45 minutes + overnight

1-Pound Loaf

Ingredients:

For the sponge:

· 1 cup warm water

· ½ cup all-purpose flour

· ½ cup whole wheat flour

· ¼ cup rye flour

· ¼ teaspoon active dry yeast

For the final dough:

· 1 cup all-purpose flour

· 1 cup whole wheat flour

· ½ cup water at room temperature

· 2 tablespoons shelled sunflower seeds

· 1 tablespoon polenta

· 1 tablespoon ground flax seeds

· 1¾ teaspoons salt - 1½ teaspoons honey

· 1 teaspoon all-purpose flour, or as needed

18

· ½ teaspoon cornmeal, or as needed

Directions:

1. Mix all of the sponge ingredients in a large mixing bowl. Cover with plastic wrap and leave for 5-6 hours to double in size.

2.Then, stir in all the ingredients for the final dough into the bowl with a sponge. Mix for 3-4 minutes with a wooden spoon until you get a sticky dough ball. Scrape down all sides of the bowl, cover again with plastic wrap, and leave overnight.

3.Line your baking sheet with parchment and dust it with ½ teaspoon all-purpose flour and cornmeal.

4.Transfer your dough onto the floured surface and press to deflate the air. Shape into a smooth rectangle pound. Transfer it onto the prepared baking sheet, lightly dust them and cover with plastic wrap for 1 hour and 30 minutes.

5.Preheat the oven to 450° F. Put a skillet on the bottom rack and pour 1 cup of hot water into it.

6.Lightly mist the top of the pound and put it into the oven. Bake for 30-35 minutes, dampening the top of the bread every 2 minutes. Remove your bread from the oven and cool completely on a cooling rack before slicing.

Nutrition:

· Calories: 185

· Carbohydrates: 26 g

Anadama Bread

Preparation Time: 1 hour

1½-PoundLoaf

Ingredients:

· 1 package (1/4oz.) active dry yeast

· 1 tablespoon sugar

· 1 cup warm water at 80°F

· 2 large eggs

· 3 tablespoons canola oil

· 1 tablespoon molasses

· 1 teaspoon white vinegar

· 1½ cups gluten-free all-purpose baking flour

· ¾ cup cornmeal

· 1½ teaspoons Xanthan gum

· ½ teaspoon salt

Direction:

1.Grease 1 ½ x 4-inch Pound pan. Sprinkle using gluten-free flour, put aside.

2.Melt sugar and yeast in warm water. Mix the vinegar, molasses, oil, and eggs in a stand mixer's bowl with a paddle attachment. Then add Whisk, Xanthan gum, cornmeal, and flour.

3.Beat for one minute on low speed, beat for two minutes on medium speed. The dough will be softer compared to yeast bread dough that has gluten. Put in a prepped pan, use a wet spatula to smooth the top. Rise with cover for 40 minutes until the dough reaches the pan's lid in a warm place.

4.Bake for 1 minute at 375° F, then loosely cover using foil. Bake till golden brown for 1¼ -15 minutes more, turn the oven off. In an oven, leave bread for 15 minutes with the door ajar. Transfer from pan onto a wire rack. Allow cooling.

Nutrition:

· Calories: 176

· Carbohydrates: 21 g

· Cholesterol: 35 mg

· Total Fat: 5 g

· Fiber: 3 g

· Protein: 4 g

· Sodium: 120 m

Sandwich Bread

Preparation Time: 1 hour

1-Pound Loaf

Ingredients:

· 1 tablespoon active dry yeast

· 2 tablespoons sugar

· 1 cup warm fat-free milk

· 2 egg whites

· 3 tablespoons canola oil

· 1 teaspoon cider vinegar

· 2½ cups gluten-free all-purpose baking flour

· 2½ teaspoons Xanthan gum

· 1 teaspoon unflavored gelatin

· ½ teaspoon salt

Direction:

1.Oil a pound pan, 9x5 inches in size, and dust with gluten-free flour reserve.

2.In warm milk, melt sugar and yeast in a small bowl—mix yeast mixture, vinegar, oil, and eggs in a stand with a paddle. Slowly whip in salt, gelatin, Xanthan gum, and flour. Whip for a minute on low speed. Whip for 2 minutes on moderate. The dough will become softer compared to the yeast bread dough that has gluten. Turn onto the prepped pan. Using a wet spatula, smoothen the surface. Put a cover and rise in a warm area for 25 minutes until dough extends to the pan top.

3.Bake for 1 minute at 375° F, loosely cover with foil. Bake till golden brown for 5 to 15 minutes more. Take out from pan onto a wire rack to let cool.

Nutrition:

· Calories: 195

· Carbohydrates: 17 g

· Cholesterol: 27 mg

· Total Fat: 4 g

· Fiber: 2 g

· Protein: 4 g

· Sodium: 120 mg

Rosemary Bread

Preparation Time: 10 minutes

1½- Pound Loaf

Ingredients:

· 1 ¼ cups warm water

· ¼ cup olive oil

· 2 egg whites

· 1 tablespoon apple cider vinegar

· ½ teaspoon baking powder

· 2 teaspoons dry active yeast

· 2 tablespoons granulated sugar

· ½ teaspoon Italian seasoning

· ¼ teaspoon ground black pepper

· 1¼ teaspoons dried rosemary

· 2 cups gluten-free almond flour / or any other gluten-free flour, leveled

· 1 cup tapioca/potato starch, leveled

· 2 teaspoons Xanthan Gum

· 1 teaspoon salt

Directions:

1.According to your bread machine manufacturer, place all the ingredients into the bread machine's greased pan.

2.Select basic cycle/standard cycle/bake/quick bread/white bread setting, then choose crust colour either medium or Light and press start to bake bread.

3.In the last kneading cycle, check the dough, it should be wet but thick, not like traditional bread dough. If the dough is too wet, put more flour, one tablespoon at a time, or until dough slightly firm.

4.When the cycle is finished, and the baker machine turns off, remove baked bread from pan and cool on wire rack.

Nutrition:

· Calories: 180

· Total fat: 3 g

· Protein:6g

· Cholesterol: 5 mg

· Sodium: 240 mg

· Carbohydrates: 24 g

· Fiber: 1 g

Flax and Sunflower Seeds Bread

Preparation Time: 10 minutes

2-Pound Loaf

Ingredients:

· 1¼ cups warm water

· ¼ cup olive oil

· 2 egg whites

· 1 tablespoon apple cider vinegar

· ½ teaspoon baking powder

· 2 teaspoons dry active yeast

· 2 tablespoons granulated sugar

· 2 cups gluten-free almond flour / or any other gluten-free flour, leveled

· 1 cup tapioca/potato starch, leveled

· 2 teaspoons Xanthan Gum

· 1 teaspoon salt

· ½ cup flax seeds

· ½ cup sunflower seeds

Directions:

1.According to your bread machine manufacturer, place all the ingredients into the bread machine's greased pan except sunflower seeds.

2.Select basic cycle/standard cycle/bake/quick bread/white bread setting, then select crust colour either medium or light and press start.

3.In the last kneading cycle, check the dough, it should be wet but thick, not like traditional bread dough. If the dough is too wet, put more flour, one tablespoon at a time, or until the dough slightly firm.

4.Add sunflower seeds 5 minutes before the kneading cycle ends.

5.When the cycle is finished and the machine turns off, remove baked bread from pan and cool on wire rack.

Nutrition:

· Calories: 190

· Total fat: 2g

· Cholesterol: 5 mg

· Sodium: 240 mg

· Carbohydrates: 21 g

· Fiber: 2 g

· Protein: 4 g

Italian Parmesan Cheese Bread

Preparation Time: 10 minutes

2-Pound Loaf

Inredients:

· 1¼ cups warm water

· ¼ cup olive oil

· 2 egg whites

· 1 tablespoon apple cider vinegar

· ½ teaspoon baking powder

· 2 teaspoons dry active yeast

· 2 tablespoons granulated sugar

· 2 cups gluten-free almond flour / or any other gluten-free flour, leveled

· 1 cup tapioca/potato starch, leveled

· 2 teaspoons Xanthan Gum

· ¼ cup grated Parmesan cheese

· 1 teaspoon salt

· 1 teaspoon Italian seasoning

· 1 teaspoon garlic powder

Directions:

1.According to your bread machine manufacturer, place all the ingredients into the bread machine's greased pan, and select a basic cycle/standard cycle/bake/quick bread/white bread setting. Then choose crust colour, either medium or light, and press start to bake bread.

2.In the last kneading cycle, check the dough, it should be wet but thick, not like traditional bread dough. If the dough is too wet, put more flour, one tablespoon at a time, or until the dough slightly firm.

3.When the cycle is finished and the machine turns off, remove baked bread from pan and cool on wire rack.

Nutrition:

· Calories: 190

· Total fat: 2 g

· Cholesterol: 2 mg

· Sodium: 240 mg

· Carbohydrates: 15 g

· Fiber: 1 g

· Protein: 2 g

Cheese & Herb Bread

Preparation Time: 10 minutes

2-Pound Loaf

Ingredients:

· 1¼ cups warm water

· ¼ cup olive oil

· 2 egg whites

· 1 tablespoon apple cider vinegar

· ½ teaspoon baking powder

· 2 teaspoons dry active yeast

· 2 tablespoons granulated sugar

· 2 cups gluten-free almond flour / or any other gluten-free flour, leveled

· 1 cup Tapioca/potato starch, leveled

· 2 teaspoons Xanthan Gum

· 1 teaspoon salt

· 2 tablespoons grated Parmesan cheese

· 1 teaspoon dried marjoram

· ¾ teaspoon dried basil

Directions:

1.According to your bread machine manufacturer, place all the ingredients into the bread machine's greased pan, and select a basic cycle/standard cycle/bake/quick bread/white bread setting. Then choose crust colour, either medium or light, and press start to bake bread.

2.In the last kneading cycle, check the dough, it should be wet but thick, not like traditional bread dough. If the dough is too wet, put more flour, one tablespoon at a time, or until the dough slightly firm.

3.When the cycle is finished and the machine turns off, remove baked bread from pan and cool on wire rack.

Nutrition:

· Calories: 230

· Total fat: 3 g

· Cholesterol: 5 mg

· Sodium: 245 mg

· Carbohydrates: 19 g

· Fiber: 1 g

· Protein: 4 g

Cinnamon Raisin Bread

Preparation Time: 15 minutes

2-Pound Loaf

Ingredients:

· 1¼ cups warm water

· ¼ cup olive oil

· 2 tablespoons honey

· 2 egg whites

· 1 tablespoon apple cider vinegar

· ½ teaspoon baking powder

· 2 teaspoons dry active yeast

· 2 tablespoons granulated sugar

· 2 cups gluten-free almond flour / or any other gluten-free flour, leveled

· 1 cup Tapioca/potato starch, leveled

· 2 teaspoons Xanthan Gum

· 1 teaspoon salt

· 1 teaspoon ground cinnamon

· 1 cup raisins

Directions:

1.According to your bread machine manufacturer, place all the ingredients into the bread machine's greased pan except raisins.

2.Select basic cycle/standard cycle/bake/quick bread/sweet bread setting, then choose crust colour either medium or Light and press start to bake bread.

3.In the last kneading cycle, check the dough, it should be wet but thick, not like traditional bread dough. If the dough is too wet, put more flour, one tablespoon at a time, or until dough slightly firm.

4.Add raisins 5 minutes before the kneading cycle ends.

5.When the cycle is finished and the machine turns off, remove baked bread from pan and cool on wire rack.

Nutrition:

· Calories: 219

· Fat: 1 g

· Cholesterol: 2 mg

· Sodium: 240 mg

· Carbohydrates: 22 g

Bakers Bread

Preparation Time: 1 hour

1-Pound Loaf

Ingredients:

· Pinch of salt

· 4 tablespoons light cream cheese softened

· ½ teaspoon cream of tartar

· 4 eggs, yolks, and whites separated

Directions:

1.Heat 2 racks in the middle of the oven at 350° F.

2.Line 2 baking pan with parchment paper, then grease with cooking spray.

3.Separate egg yolks from the whites and place them in separate mixing bowls.

4.Beat the egg whites and cream of tartar with a hand mixer until stiff, about 3 to 5 minutes. Do not over-beat.

5.Whisk the cream cheese, salt, and egg yolks until smooth.

6.Slowly fold the cheese mix into the whites until fluffy.

7.Spoon ¼ cup measure of the batter onto the baking sheets, 6 mounds on each sheet.

8.Bake in the oven for 1 to 22 minutes, alternating racks halfway through.

9. Cool and serve.

Nutrition:

· Calories: 191

· Fat: 3.2 g

· Carbohydrates:1 g

· Protein: 2.4 g

· Sodium: 30 mg

Bulgur Bread

Preparation Time: 15 minutes

1½-Pound Loaf

Ingredients:

· ½ cup bulgur

· 1/3 cup boiling water

· 1 egg

· 1 cup water

· 1 tablespoon butter

· 1½ tablespoons milk powder

· 1 tablespoon sugar

· 2 teaspoons salt

· 3¼ cup flour

· 1 teaspoon dried yeast

Directions:

1.Bulgur pour boiling water into a small container and cover with a lid. Leave to stand for 30 minutes.

2.Cut butter into small cubes.

3.Stir the egg with water in a measuring container. The total volume of eggs with water should be 300 ml.

4.Put all the ingredients in the bread maker in the order that is described in the instructions for your bread maker. Bake in the basic mode, medium crust.

Nutrition:

· Calories: 255

· Carbohydrates: 3 g

· Fats: 3 g

· Protein: 1½ g

· Sodium: 480 mg

· Fiber: 1.2 g

Almond Meal Bread

Preparation Time: 1 hour

1-Pound Loaf

Ingredients:

· 4 eggs, pasteurized

· ¼ cup melted coconut oil

· 1 tablespoon apple cider vinegar

· 2¼ cups almond meal

· 1 teaspoon baking soda

· ¼ cup ground flaxseed meal

· 1 teaspoon onion powder

· 1 tablespoon minced garlic

· 1 teaspoon of sea salt

· 1 teaspoon chopped sage leaves

· 1 teaspoon fresh thyme

· 1 teaspoon chopped rosemary leaves

Directions:

1.Gather all the ingredients for the bread and plug in the bread machine having the capacity of 2 pounds of bread recipe.

2.Take a large bowl, crack eggs in it and then beat in coconut oil and vinegar until well blended.

3. Take a separate large bowl, place the almond meal in it, add remaining ingredients, and stir until well mixed.

4.Add egg mixture into the bread bucket, top with flour mixture, shut the lid, select the "basic/white" cycle or "low-carb" setting and then press the up/down arrow button to adjust baking time according to your bread machine; it will take 3 to 4 hours.

5.Then press the crust button to select light crust if available, and press the "start/stop" button to switch on the bread machine.

6.When the bread machine beeps, open the lid, then take out the bread basket and lift out the bread.

7.Let bread cool on a wire rack for 1 hour, then cut it into ten pounds and serve.

Nutrition:

· Calories: 194

· Sodium: 240 mg

· Fat: 2 g

· Protein: 4 g

· Carbohydrates: 2.1 g

· Fiber: 2 g

· Net Carbohydrates: 0.3 g

Italian Blue Cheese Bread

Preparation Time: 3 hours

1½-Pound Loaf

Ingredients:

· 1 teaspoon dry yeast

· 2½ cups almond flour

· 1½ teaspoon salt

· 1 tablespoon sugar

· 1 tablespoon olive oil

· ½ cup blue cheese

· 1 cup water

Directions:

1.Mix all the ingredients.

2.Start baking.

3.When the cycle is finished and the machine turns off, remove baked bread from pan and cool on wire rack.

Nutrition:

· Calories: 194

· Carbohydrates 5 g

· Fats 4.6 g

· Protein: 6 g

· Fiber: 1.5 g

· Sodium: 360 mg

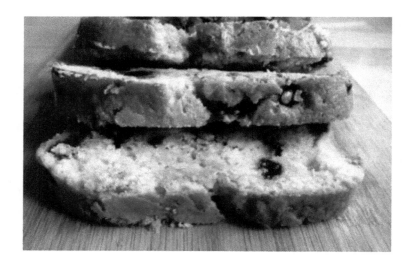

Macadamia Nut Bread

Preparation Time: 10 minutes

1½-Pound Loaf

Ingredients:

· 1 cup / 135 grams macadamia nuts

· 5 eggs, pasteurized

· 1 cup water

· ½ teaspoon apple cider vinegar

· ¼ cup / 30 grams coconut flour

· ½ teaspoon baking soda

Directions:

1.Gather all the ingredients for the bread and plug in the bread machine having the capacity of 1 pound of bread recipe.

2.Place nuts in a blender, pulse for 2 to 3 minutes until mixture reaches a consistency of butter, and then blend in eggs and vinegar until smooth.

3.Stir in flour and baking soda until well mixed.

4.Add the batter into the bread bucket, shut the lid, select the "basic/white" cycle or "low-carb" setting and then press the up/down arrow button to adjust baking time according to your bread machine; it will take 3 to 4 hours.

5.Then press the crust button to select light crust if available, and press the "start/stop" button to switch on the bread machine.

6.When the bread machine beeps, open the lid, then take out the bread basket and lift out the bread.

7.Let bread cool on a wire rack for 1 hour, then cut it into eight pounds and serve.

Nutrition:

· Calories: 175

· Sodium: 20 mg

· Fat: 1.3 g

· Protein: 5.6 g

· Carbohydrates: 3.9 g

· Fiber: 3 g

· Net Carbohydrates: 0.9 g

Cheesy Garlic Bread

Preparation Time: 1 hour

2-Pound Loaf

Ingredients:

For the Bread:

· 5 eggs, pasteurized

· 1 cup water

· 2 cups / 10 grams almond flour

· ½ teaspoon Xanthan gum

· 1 teaspoon garlic powder

· 1 teaspoon salt

· 1 teaspoon parsley

· 1 teaspoon Italian seasoning

· 1 teaspoon dried oregano

· 1 stick of butter, grass-fed, unsalted, melted

· 1 cup grated mozzarella cheese

· 2 tablespoons ricotta cheese

· 1 cup / 235 grams grated cheddar cheese

· 1/3 cup / 30 grams grated parmesan cheese

For the Topping:

· ½ stick of butter, grass-fed, unsalted, melted

· 1 teaspoon garlic powder

Directions:

1.Gather all the ingredients for the bread and plug in the bread machine having the capacity of 2 pounds of bread recipe.

2.Take a large bowl, crack eggs in it and then whisk until blended.

3.Take a separate large bowl, place flour in it, and stir in Xanthan gum and all the cheeses until well combined.

4.Take a medium bowl, place butter in it, add all the seasonings in it, and stir until mixed.

5.Add egg mixture into the bread bucket, top with seasoning mixture and flour mixture, shut the lid, select the "basic/white" cycle or "low-carb" setting and then press the up/down arrow button to adjust baking time according to your bread machine; it will take 3 to 4 hours.

6.Then press the crust button to select light crust if available, and press the "start/stop" button to switch on the bread machine.

7.When the bread machine beeps, open the lid, then take out the bread basket and lift out the bread.

8.Prepare the topping by mixing together melted butter and garlic powder and brush the mixture on top of the bread.

9.Let bread cool on a wire rack for 1 hour, then cut it into sixteen pounds and serve.

Nutrition:

· Calories: 250

· Fat: 1.5 g

· Sodium: 400 mg

· Protein: 7.2 g

· Carbohydrates: 3 g

· Fiber: 1.6 g

· Net Carbohydrates: 1.4 g

Almond Pumpkin Quick Bread

Preparation Time: 35 minutes

1½-Pound Loaf

Ingredients

· 1/3 cup vegetable oil

· ½ cup water

· 3 large eggs

· 1 ½ cups pumpkin puree, canned

· 1 cup granulated sugar

· 1½ teaspoons baking powder

· ½ teaspoon baking soda

· ¼ teaspoon salt

· ¾ teaspoon ground cinnamon

· ¼ teaspoon ground nutmeg

· ¼ teaspoon ground ginger

· 3 cups almond flour

· ½ cup chopped pecans

Directions

1.Spray your bread machine pan with cooking spray.

2.In a bowl, mix all the wet ingredients until blended. Add all the dry ingredients except pecans until mixed.

3.Pour the batter onto your bread machine pan and place it back inside the bread machine. Close the cover securely.

4.Turn on the bread machine and select QUICK BREAD cycle then press START.

5.When your bread machine pings, pause and open the lid then add the chopped pecans. Then close the lid and press START to let the cycle continue.

6.Once cycle is finished, loosen the pound from the pan and transfer to a cooling rack.

7.Slice and serve with your favorite keto soup.

Nutrition:

· Calories: 250

· Sodium: 70 mg

· Fat: 1.5 g

· Protein: 7.2 g

· Carbohydrates: 3 g

· Fiber: 1.6 g

· Net Carbohydrates: 1.4 g

Keto Basil Parmesan Slices

Preparation Time: 10 minutes

Cooking Time: 2 hour s

1½-Pound loaf

Ingredients:

· 1 cup water

· ½ cup parmesan cheese, grated

· 3 tablespoons sugar

· 1 tablespoon dried basil

· 1½ tablespoons olive oil

· 1 teaspoon salt

· 3 cups almond flour

· 2 teaspoons active dry yeast

Directions:

1.Place all the ingredients in your bread machine pan according to the list stated in the ingredients list.

2.Close the lid then set the bread machine on BASIC cycle and press START.

3.Once the cycle is done, move pound to a cooling rack.

4.Slice and serve as a side dish for your soup or main course.

Nutrition:

· Calories: 250

· Sodium: 240 mg

· Fat: 1.5 g

· Protein: 7.2 g

· Carbohydrates: 3 g

· Fiber: 1.6 g

· Net Carbohydrates: 1.4 g

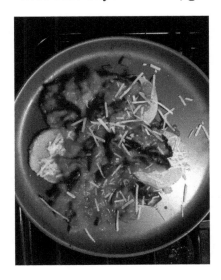

Onion Bread

Preparation Time: 45 minutes

2-Pound Loaf

Ingredients:

· 1½ cups water

· 2 tablespoons + 2 teaspoons butter, unsalted

· 1½ teaspoons salt

· 1 tablespoon + 1 teaspoon sugar

· 2 tablespoons + 2 teaspoons non-fat dry milk

· 4 cups almond flour

· 2 teaspoons active dry yeast

· 4 tablespoons dry onion soup mix

Directions:

1.Add all ingredients except dry onion mix in the bread machine pan according to the list above.

2.Close the lid cover. Select BASIC cycle on your bread machine and then press START.

3.Your machine will ping after around 30 to 40 minutes. This is your signal to add whatever fruit, nut, or flavoring you wish to add to your dough. Pause your bread machine and add the dry onion soup mix.

4.Press START again and allow the cycle to continue.

5.Once your pound is finished, transfer it to a cooling rack.

6. Slice and serve with cream cheese or butter or as a soup side dish.

Nutrition:

· Calories: 250

· Sodium: 360 mg

· Fat: 1.5 g Protein: 7.2 g

· Carbohydrates: 3 g

· Fiber: 1.6 g

Sundried Tomato Quick Bread

Preparation Time: 25 minutes

1½-Pound Loaf

Ingredients :

· 2¼ cups almond flour

· ½ water

· 1 tablespoon baking powder

· 1 teaspoon kosher salt

· 3 large eggs

· 1½ cups buttermilk

· 6 tablespoons canola oil

· 1 tablespoon dried basil

· 1 cup sundried tomato roughly chopped

Directions:

1.Place all the ingredients in your bread machine bucket except for basil and sundried tomato.

2.Secure the lid cover. Select the QUICK BREAD setting on your bread machine then press START.

3.Wait for the ping or the fruit and nut signal to open the lid and add the basil and sundried tomato. Close the lid again and press START to continue.

4.When the cycle finishes, transfer the pound to a wire rack and let it cool.

5. Slice and serve.

Nutrition:

· Calories: 250

· Sodium: 230 mg

· Fat: 1.5 g

· Protein: 7.2 g

· Carbohydrates: 3 g

· Fiber: 1.6 g

· Net Carbohydrates: 1.4 g

Cheddar Bacon and Chive Bread

Preparation Time: 10 minutes

1½-Pound Loaf

Ingredients

· 2¼ cups almond flour

· ½ water

· 1 tablespoon baking powder

· 1 teaspoon kosher salt

· 3 large eggs

· 1½ cups buttermilk

· 6 tablespoons canola oil

· 3 tablespoons finely chopped chives

· 1 cup shredded cheddar sharp cheese

· 6 strips bacon cook and crumbled

Directions:

1.Place all the ingredients in your bread machine bucket pan except for bacon.

2.Close the cover. Select the QUICK BREAD setting on your bread machine then press START.

3.Wait for the fruit and nut signal. Pause and open the lid and add the bacon. Close the lid again and press START to continue.

4.When the cycle finishes, transfer the pound to a wire rack and let it cool.

5.Slice and serve.

Nutrition:

· Calories: 250

· Sodium: 270 mg

· Fat: 1.5 g

· Protein: 7.2 g

· Carbohydrates: 3 g

· Fiber: 1.6 g

· Net Carbohydrates: 1.4 g

Keto Tortilla Wraps

Preparation Time: 50 minutes

1-Pound Loaf

Ingredients

· 1 cup golden flaxseed meal

· 2 tablespoons coconut flour

· ½ teaspoon Xanthan gum

· ½ teaspoon salt

· 1 tablespoon butter

· 1 cup warm water

Directions

1.Add all ingredients into your bread machine. Close the lid cover.

2.Select DOUGH cycle and press START.

3.Once the cycle is finished, remove the dough and transfer it to a lightly floured working table.

4.Divide the dough into equal chunks. Roll out the dough into a thin shape.

5.On a skillet over low heat, cook the tortilla for 1-2 minutes each tortilla. Remove from the skillet and cover with a towel. The tortillas should be soft and not stiff.

6.Serve with your favorite filling.

Nutrition:

· Calories: 250

· Sodium: 130 mg

· Fat: 1.5 g

· Protein: 7.2 g

· Carbohydrates: 3 g

· Fiber: 1.6 g

· Net Carbohydrates: 1.4 g

Keto Southern Biscuit

Preparation Time: 2 hours 15 minutes

5- Biscuits

Ingredients :

· 2/3 cup milk

· ½ cup water

· 2 large eggs, lightly beaten

· 1/3 cup butter, unsalted and softened

· 1 tablespoon honey

· 1¼ teaspoons salt

· 3½ cups almond flour

· 3 teaspoons active dry yeast

Directions:

1.Place all the ingredients according to the list arrangement above. Close the bread machine lid.

2.On your bread machine, select DOUGH cycle then press the START button.

3.Once the cycle ends, remove the dough and transfer it to a floured working table. Roll out the dough until it is ½-inch thick.

4.Cut into 5sizes and arrange on a greased baking sheet. Let it rise for an hour.

5.Preheat your oven to 425° F.

6. Pop the baking sheet into the oven and bake for 15 minutes or until lightly golden.

7.Serve with your favorite soup or fill with your favorite meat filling.

Nutrition:

· Calories: 250

· Sodium: 360 mg

· Fat: 1.5 g

· Protein: 7.2 g

· Carbohydrates:3g

· Net Carbohydrates: 1.4 g

· Fiber: 1.6 g

Cloud Bread

Preparation Time: 50 minutes

1-Pound Loaf

Ingredients:

· 3 oz. cream cheese, full-fat and softened

· ¼ cup water

· ½ teaspoon salt

· 3 large eggs

· ¼ teaspoon cream of tartar

· electric blender

· standard sized flat sheet

Directions:

1.Adjust the temperature of the stove to heat at 300° F.

2.Layer a flat sheet with baking lining and set to the side.

3.Divide the whites and yolks of the eggs into two different dishes.

4.Blend the salt and cream cheese with the yolks with an electric blender.

5.Combine the cream of tartar with the whites of the eggs and pulse with the electric blender for approximately 4 minutes until firm.

6.Blend the two dishes together and be sure not to over mix.

7.Evenly distribute the batter into 6 sections on the prepped flat sheet.

8.Slightly press each mound to flatten to your desired thickness.

9.Heat for approximately half an hour and distribute to a wire rack.

10. Enjoy immediately with a half tablespoon of butter

Nutrition:

· Calories: 225

· Carbohydrates: 5 g

· Protein: 4 g

· Fat: 7 g

· Net Carbohydrates: 0.6 g

· Sugar: 0 g

· Sodium: 120 mg

Pumpkin Pecan Bread

Preparation Time: 10 minutes

1¼ Pound Loaf

Ingredients:

· ½ cup milk

· ½ cup canned pumpkin

· 1 egg

· 2 tablespoons margarine or butter, cut up

· 3 cups bread flour

· 3 tablespoons packed brown sugar

· ¾ teaspoon salt

· ¼ teaspoon ground nutmeg

· ¼ teaspoon ground ginger

· 1½ teaspoons ground cloves

· 1 teaspoon active dry yeast or bread machine yeast

· ¾ cup coarsely chopped pecans

Directions:

1.Add all ingredients to the machine pan.

2.Select the basic cycle.

3.When the cycle is finished and the machine turns off, remove baked bread from pan and cool on wire rack.

Nutrition:

· Calories: 189

· Fat: 6 g

· Cholesterol: 1 mg

· Sodium: 186 mg

· Carbohydrates: 23 g

· Fiber: 4 g

· Protein: 4 g

Ricotta Chive Bread

Preparation Time: 10 minutes

1-Pound Loaf

Ingredients:

· 1 cup lukewarm water

· 1/3 cup whole or part-skim ricotta cheese

· 1½ teaspoons salt

· 1 tablespoon granulated sugar

· 3 cups bread flour

· ½ cup chopped chives

· 2½ teaspoons instant yeast

Directions:

1.Add ingredients to bread machine pan except for dried fruit.

2.Choose a basic bread setting and light/medium crust.

Nutrition:

· Calories:192

· Sodium: 370 mg

· Total Fat: 0 g

· Cholesterol: 2 mg

· Sodium: 360 mg

· Carbohydrates: 17 g

· Fiber: 1 g

· Protein: 3 g

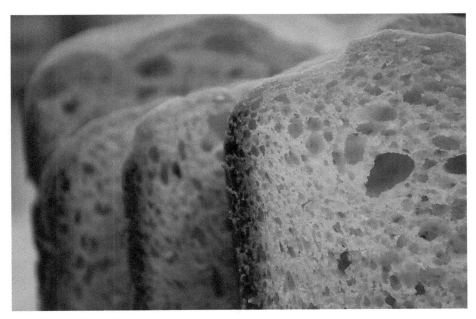

Red Hot Cinnamon Bread

Preparation Time: 1 hour

1-Pound Loaf

Ingredients

· ¼ cup lukewarm water

· ½ cup lukewarm milk

· ¼ cup softened butter

· 2¼ teaspoons instant yeast

· 1¼ teaspoons salt

· ¼ cup sugar

· 1 teaspoon vanilla

· 1 large egg, lightly beaten

· 3 cups all-purpose flour

· ½ cup Cinnamon Red Hot candies

Directions

1.Add ingredients to bread machine pan except for candy.

2.Choose dough setting.

3.After the cycle is over, turn the dough out into a bowl and cover, let rise for 45 minutes to one hour.

4.Gently punch down the dough and shape it into a rectangle.

5. Knead in the cinnamon candies in 1/3 at a time.

6.Shape the dough into a pound and place in a greased or parchment-lined pound pan.

7.Tent the pan loosely with lightly greased plastic wrap, and allow a second rise for 40-50 minutes.

8.Preheat oven 350° F.

9.Bake 30-40 minutes.

10.Remove and cool on wire rack before slicing.

Nutrition:

· Calories: 187

· Total Fat: 6.9 g

· Cholesterol: 18 mg

· Sodium: 367 mg

· Carbohydrates: 30 g

· Fiber: 1 g

· Protein: 4.6 g

Cheddar Olive Loaf

Preparation Time: 15 Minutes

1-Pound Loaf

Ingredients

· 1 cup water room temperature

· 4 teaspoons sugar

· ¾ teaspoon salt

· 1¼ cups shredded sharp cheddar cheese

· 3 cups bread flour

· 2 teaspoons active dry yeast

· ¾ cup pimiento olives, drained and sliced

Directions

1.Add all ingredients except olives to the machine pan.

2.Select basic bread setting.

3. At prompt before second knead, mix in olives.

Nutrition:

· Calories: 164

- Total Fat: 4 g (2 g sat. fat)

- Cholesterol: 9 mg

- Sodium: 299 mg

- Carbohydrates: 19 g

- Fiber: 1 g

- Protein: 5 g

Wild Rice Cranberry Bread

Preparation Time: 25 minutes

1½-Pound Loaf

Ingredients:

· 1¼ cups water

· ¼ cup skim milk powder

· 1¼ teaspoons salt

· 2 tablespoons liquid honey

· 1 tablespoon extra-virgin olive oil

· 3 cup all-purpose flour

· ¾ cup cooked wild rice

· ¼ cup pine nuts

· ¾teaspoons celery seeds

· 1½ teaspoons freshly ground black pepper

· 1 teaspoon bread machine or instant yeast

· 2/3 cup dried cranberries

Directions

1.Add all ingredients to the machine pan except the cranberries.

2.Place pan into the oven chamber.

3.Select basic bread setting.

4. At the signal to add ingredients, add in the cranberries.

Nutrition:

· Calories: 225

· Total Fat: 7.1 g

· Cholesterol: 5 mg

· Sodium: 322 mg

· Carbohydrates: 33 g

· Fiber. 1 g

· Protein: 6.7 g

Carrot Polenta Loaf

Preparation Time: 5 minutes

Cooking Time: 3 hours

1-Pound Loaf

Ingredients:

· ½ cup lukewarm water

· 2 tablespoons extra-virgin olive oil

· 1 teaspoons salt

· 1½ tablespoons sugar

· 1½ tablespoons dried thyme

· 1½ cups freshly-grated carrots

· ½ cup yellow cornmeal

· 1 cup light rye flour

· 2½ cups bread flour

· 3 teaspoons instant active dry yeast

Directions:

1.Add all ingredients to the machine pan.

2.Select dough setting.

3.When the cycle is complete, turn dough onto lightly floured surface.

4.Knead the dough and shape it into an oval; cover with plastic wrap and let rest for 5 to 15 minutes.

5. After resting, turn bottom side up and flatten.

6.Fold the top 1/3 of the way to the bottom. Then fold the bottom a 1/3 of the way over the top. Press dough with the palm of your hand to make an indent in the center, then fold the top completely down to the bottom, sealing the seam.

7.Preheat oven 400.

8.Dust a baking sheet with cornmeal, place dough on and cover in a warm place to rise for 1 minute.

9.After rising, make 3 deep diagonal slashes on the top and brush the top of the bread with cold water.

10. Bake for 1 to 25 minutes or until nicely browned

Nutrition:

· Calories: 220

· Total Fat: 2 g

· Cholesterol: 1 mg

· Sodium: 366 mg

· Carbohydrates: 27 g

· Fiber: 2g

Cheese Cauliflower Broccoli Bread

Preparation Time: 10 minutes

1-Pound Loaf

Ingredients:

· ¼ cup water

· 4 tablespoons oil

· 1 egg white

· 1 teaspoon lemon juice

· 2/3 cup grated cheddar cheese

· 3 tablespoons green onion

· ½ cup broccoli, chopped

· ½ cup cauliflower, chopped

· ½ teaspoon lemon-pepper seasoning

· 2 cups bread flour

· 1 teaspoon regular or quick-rising yeast

Directions

1.Add all ingredients to the machine pan.

2.Select basic bread setting.

3.When the cycle is finished and the machine turns off, remove baked bread from pan and cool on wire rack.

Nutrition:

· Calories: 196

· Total Fat: 7.4 g

· Cholesterol: 1½ mg

· Sodium: 56 mg

· Carbohydrates: 17 g

· Protein: 4.9 g

Orange Cappuccino Bread

Preparation Time: 5 minutes

1-Pound Loaf

Ingredients

· 1 cup water

· 1 tablespoon instant coffee granules

· 2 tablespoons butter or margarine, softened

· 1 teaspoon grated orange peel

· 3 cups bread flour

· 2 tablespoons dry milk

· ¼ cup sugar

· 1¼ teaspoons salt

· 2¼ teaspoons bread machine or quick active dry yeast

Directions

1.Add all ingredients to machine pan.

2.Select basic bread setting.

Nutrition:

· Calories: 175

· Total Fat: 2 g

· Cholesterol: 5 mg

· Sodium: 300 mg

· Carbohydrates: 31 g

· Fiber: 1 g

· Protein: 4 g

Celery Bread

Preparation Time: 10 minutes

1-Pound Loaf

Ingredients:

· 1 cup(5oz.) can cream of celery soup

· 3 tablespoons low-fat milk, heated

· 1 tablespoon vegetable oil

· 1¼ teaspoons celery, garlic, or onion salt

· ¾ cup celery, fresh/sliced thin

· 1 tablespoon celery leaves, fresh, chopped -optional

· 1 egg

· 3 cups bread flour

· ¼ teaspoon sugar

· ¼ teaspoon ginger

· ½ cup quick-cooking oats

· 2 tablespoons gluten

· 2 teaspoons celery seeds

· 1 package active dry yeast

Directions:

1.Add all ingredients to machine pan.

2.Select basic bread setting.

3. When the cycle is finished and the machine turns off, remove baked bread from pan and cool on wire rack.

Nutrition:

· Calories: 183

· Total Fat: 3.6 g

· Cholesterol: 55 mg

· Sodium: 366 mg

· Carbohydrates: 1½ g

· Fiber: 0 g

· Protein: 2.6 g

Anise Almond Bread

Preparation Time: 2 5 minutes

1-Pound Loaf

Ingredients:

· ¾ cup water

· 1 or ¼ cup egg substitute

· ¼ cup butter or margarine, softened

· ¼ cup sugar

· ½ teaspoon salt

· 3 cups bread flour

· 1 teaspoon anise seed

· 2 teaspoons active dry yeast

· ½ cup almonds, chopped small

Directions:

1.Add all ingredients to the machine pan except almonds.

2.Select basic bread setting.

3.After prompt, add almonds.

Nutrition:

· Calories: 202

· Total Fat: 4 g

· Cholesterol: 4 mg

· Sodium: 124 mg

· Carbohydrates: 7 g

· Fiber: 0 g

· Protein: 3 g

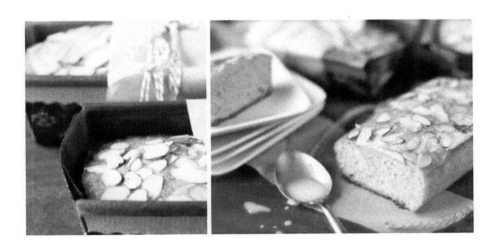

Coffee Cake Muffins

Preparation Time: 1 hour

1½-Pound Loaf

Difficulty : Intermediate

Ingredients :

For the bread :

· 2 tablespoons butter softened

· 2 ounces cream cheese softened

· 1 teaspoon baking powder

· ¼ cup teaspoon salt

· 1/3 cup Swerve

· 2 teaspoon vanilla

· ½ cup unsweetened almond milk

· 1 cup almond flour

· ½ cup coconut flour

· 4 eggs

For the topping:

· 1 teaspoon cinnamon

· 2 tablespoons coconut flour

- ¼ cup Swerve

- ¼ cup butter softened

- 1 cup almond flour

Directions:

1.Preheat oven to 355º F. Line a muffin tin with paper liners or grease the muffin tin.

2.Place cream cheese, vanilla, and eggs in a food processor and blend until well combined.

3.Put the dry ingredients in a big bowl and thoroughly mix.

4.Combine the dry and wet ingredients and whisk.

5.For the topping, add your ingredients together in a separate bowl and mix.

6.Bake 25 minutes until golden. When you insert a toothpick, it should come out clean.

Nutrition:

- Calories: 222

- Total Fat: 11 g

- Cholesterol: 72 mg

- Sodium:156 mg

- Protein: 7 g

Chocolate Chip Muffins

Preparation Time: 1 hour

1-Pound Loaf

Difficulty : Intermediate

Ingredients:

· 1 cup almond flour

· 2 large eggs

· 1 teaspoon baking powder

· ¼ cup Erythritol

· 40 g butter (melted)

· 40 ml unsweetened almond milk

· 1 teaspoon vanilla extract

· 50 g (Unsweetened) dark chocolate

Directions:

1.Preheat your oven to a temperature of 350° F.Line your 13.75"x 1 1.45" muffin pan with cupcake liners or grease it.

2.Mix the almond flour and the baking powder together in a bowl.

3.Add 2 eggs into the bowl and stir to mix. Melt the butter then add it into the bowl.

4.Add the other ingredients (apart from the chocolate) and whisk.

5. Spoon the batter into your muffin tray filling it up to a level of ¾.

6.Cut the pieces of chocolate into thin pounds. Pierce them through the top of the muffins.

7.Bake for 1 minute. A toothpick should come out clean when poked through the muffin.

8.Let them cool for 5minutes.

Nutrition:

· Calories: 229

· Fat: 1½ g

· Saturated

· Fat: 2g

· Protein: 7g

· Carbohydrates: 11g

· Sodium: 96 mg

· Fiber: 0g

· Sodium: 30 mg

· Sugar: 2g

Pumpkin Muffins

Preparation Time: 1 hour

2-Pound Loaf

Difficulty : Beginner

Ingredients :

· 5 eggs

· ½ cup liquid coconut oil

· 2 tablespoons butter

· 1 cup pumpkin puree

· 1½ tablespoons pumpkin pie spice

· 1½ cup Swerve

· 2 teaspoons vanilla extract

· ½ cup coconut flour

· 1 teaspoon salt

· 1½ teaspoons baking powder

Filling

· 2 ounces cream cheese

· 2 tablespoons heavy whipping cream

· 1 tablespoon swerve or sweetener of your choice

· 1 teaspoon vanilla extract

Directions:

1.Preheat oven to 350° F then grease the 15.75" x 11.25"muffin pan or line it with muffin liners.

2.Melt the butter.

3.Add eggs, coconut oil, melted butter, pumpkin puree, pumpkin pie spice, swerve and vanilla extract to a large bowl and mix until well combined.

4.Add coconut flour, salt, and baking powder to the other ingredients and mix.

5.Scoop batter into prepared muffin tins, filling each one ¾ way.

6.In another bowl, add the ingredients for the filling and stir until well combined and smooth.

7.Place 1 tsp of filling in the center of each muffin.

8.Using a toothpick swirl cream cheese batter into the muffin

9.Bake for 1 minute.

Notes: These muffins need a thicker batter than most muffins do.

Nutrition:

· Calories: 221

· Carbohydrates: 3 g

· Protein: 2 g

Banana Bread Muffins

Preparation Time: 1 hour

2-Pound Loaf

Difficulty : Beginner

Ingredients :

· ¼ cup Erythritol sweetener, confectioner

· ¾ cup almond flour

· 3 tablespoons butter, unsalted and melted

· ¼ cup sour cream, full-fat

· 1¼ teaspoons baking powder, gluten-free

· 4 oz. walnuts, raw and chopped

· 1/3 teaspoon ground cinnamon

· 2 teaspoons butter, unsalted, cubed, and separate

· 1½ teaspoon banana extract, sugar-free

· 2 teaspoons almond flour, separate

· ¼ cup almond milk, unsweetened

· 1 teaspoon vanilla extract, sugar-free

· 2 teaspoons Erythritol sweetener, confectioner and separate

· 1 large egg

Directions:

1.Dissolve the 3 teaspoons of butter completely in a 6.5" saucepan and set to the side.

2.Adjust the temperature of the stove to heat at 350º F. Line a small cupcake tin with 6 papers or silicone cups. Set aside.

3.Use a food blender to pulse the 2 teaspoons. of almond flour, 2 teaspoons. of butter and walnuts until a crumbly consistency. Set to the side.

4.Blend the 1/3 cup of Erythritol, cinnamon, baking powder, and ¾ cup of almond flour until incorporated fully.

5.Combine the eggs, sour cream, banana extract, almond milk, melted butter, and vanilla extract into the mixture until integrated.

6.Evenly distribute to the prepped cupcake tin and dust with the crumble from the food processor. Apply slight pressure to adhere to the batter.

7.Evenly spread the 2 teaspoons of Erythritol over the muffins.

8.Heat for a total of 1 minute and take out of the stove to the countertop.

9.Wait about half an hour before serving. Enjoy!

Nutrition:

· Calories: 211

· Carbohydrates:4 g

· Sodium: 40 mg

- Protein: 7g

- Fat: 1g

- Cholesterol: 23 mg

- Sodium: 43 mg

- Potassium: 95 mg

- Fiber: 1 g

- Sugar: 1 g

Cinnamon Muffins

Preparation Time: 1hour

1½-Pound Loaf

Difficulty : Beginner

Ingredients:

For the muffin:

· 1/3cup almond flour

· ½ teaspoon baking powder, gluten-free

· 1/3 cup almond butter

· ½ tablespoons ground cinnamon

· 5 oz. pumpkin puree

· 1/3 cup coconut oil

· 1½ cavity muffin tin or 24 cavity mini muffin tin

For the optional topping:

· ¼ cup coconut butter

· ½ tablespoon, Swerve sweetener, granulated

· ¼ cup milk

· 1 teaspoon lemon juice

Directions:

1.Set your stove to heat at the temperature of 350° F.

2.Use silicone or baking cups to line your preferred cupcake tin. Set to the side.

3.Combine the almond flour, baking powder, and cinnamon with a whisk in a glass dish. Remove any lumpiness present.

4.Blend the almond butter, pumpkin puree, and coconut oil into the mix until incorporated.

5.Evenly divide the batter between the cavities in the prepped cupcake tin.

6.Heat for approximately 13 minutes and transfer to a wire rack after waiting 5 minutes.

7.If you are applying the topping, blend the lemon juice, milk, Swerve, and coconut butter until smooth.

8.Evenly empty the topping once the muffins have completely cooled.

Nutrition:

· Calories: 329

· Fat: 9g

· Saturated Fat: 2 g

· Protein: 5g

· Carbohydrates: 1.2 g

Chocolate Muffins

Preparation Time: 1 hour

1½-Pound Loaf

Difficulty : Beginner

Ingredients :

· ½ teaspoon salt

· 2 cups almond flour, blanched

· ½ cup cocoa powder, unsweetened

· ¾ cup Pyure Stevia blend, granulated

· 1 teaspoon baking powder, gluten-free

· 4 large eggs

· ¼ cup coconut oil, melted

· 2 oz. almond milk, unsweetened

· 1 teaspoon vanilla extract, sugar-free

· 1.75 oz. dark chocolate, Stevia sweetened and chopped

Directions:

1.Set the temperature of the stove to heat at 350° F. Cover the cavities of the cupcake tin with baking liner or silicone. Set to the side.

2.Liquefy the coconut oil for approximately 3 minutes in a saucepan.

3.Chop the chocolate roughly into small chunks and set aside.

4.Blend the salt, baking powder, almond flour, Pyure Stevia blend, and cocoa powder until fully incorporated.

5.Combine the melted coconut oil, vanilla extract, almond milk, and eggs into the mix and toss until integrated.

6.Finally, incorporate the chopped chocolate into the mix.

7.Evenly divide the batter into the prepped cupcake tin.

8.For the duration of approximately 26 minutes, heat the muffins and then transfer them to the countertop.

9.Wait about 5minutes before serving and enjoy!

Nutrition:

· Calories: 229

· Sodium: 120 mg

· Protein: 7g

· Net carbohydrates: 3.5 g

· Fat: 1¼ g

Coffee Cake Muffins

Preparation Time: 1 hour

1½-Pound Loaf

Difficulty : Intermediate

Ingredients:

For the muffins:

· ½ teaspoon ground cinnamon

· 2 cups almond flour

· ½ cup almond milk, unsweetened

· 1/3 cup Swerve sweetener, granulated

· 3 tablespoons coconut flour

· ¼ teaspoon salt

· 3 teaspoons baking powder, gluten-free

· ½ cup butter, unsalted

· 4 large eggs

· ½ teaspoon vanilla extract, sugar-free

· 1½ cavity muffin tin

For the optional topping :

· ½ cup almond flour

· 3 tablespoons Sukrin Gold brown sugar substitute

· ¼ cup butter, unsalted and melted

· 2 tablespoons coconut flour

· ¾ teaspoons ground cinnamon

Directions:

1.Adjust your stove to heat at the temperature of 325° F.

2.Cover the 1 ½ cavities with silicone or baking cups and set them to the side.

3.Blend the salt, cinnamon, baking powder, coconut flour, Swerve, and almond flour in a glass dish until all lumpiness is no longer present.

4.Combine the vanilla extract, almond milk, eggs, and butter into the mix and blend until incorporated fully.

5.Equally, distribute to the prepped cupcake tin.

6.For the optional glaze, dissolve the butter in a saucepan and turn the burner off.

7.Combine the cinnamon, coconut flour, Sukrin Gold, and almond flour in a 5" round pan and evenly distribute to the top of the batter.

8. Heat in the stove for approximately half an hour and take out to place on the countertop.

9.Wait about 5minutes before serving and enjoy!

Nutrition:

· Calories: 210

· Sodium: 60 mg

· Protein: 9g

· Net carbohydrates: 3.9 g

· Fat: 24 g

· Sugar: 1 g

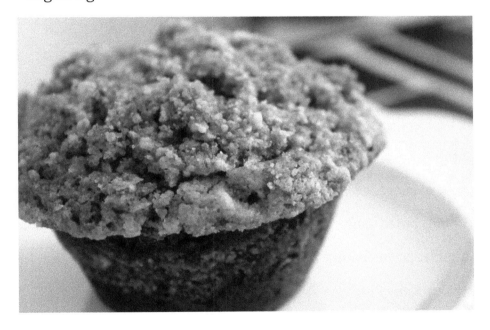

Lemon Poppyseed Muffins

Preparation Time: 1 hour

1½-Pound Loaf

Difficulty : Expert

Ingredients :

· ¼ cup golden flaxseed meal

· ¾ cup almond flour

· 1/3 cup Erythritol sweetener, granulated

· 2 tablespoons poppy seeds

· 1 tablespoon baking powder, gluten-free

· 3 large eggs

· ¼ cup butter, salted and melted

· 2 tablespoons lemon zest

· ¼ cup heavy cream

· 25 drops Stevia liquid

· 1 teaspoon vanilla extract, sugar-free

· 3 tablespoons lemon juice

Directions:

1.Liquefy the butter in a 5.5" saucepan and turn the burner off.

2.In the meantime, prepare a muffin tin with baking cups or silicone. Set to the side.

3. Heat your stove to the temperature of 350° F.

4.Combine the poppy seeds, Erythritol, flaxseed meal, and almond flour with a whisk until integrated.

5.Blend the heavy cream, eggs, and melted butter until incorporated fully.

6.Finally combine the lemon juice, vanilla extract, Stevia liquid, baking powder, and lemon zest into the mix and blend well.

7.Divide the batter equally to the prepped muffin tin and heat for approximately 1 minute.

8.Place on the countertop and wait about 5minutes before serving.

Nutrition:

· Calories: 210

· Sodium: 60 mg

· Protein: 4 g

· Net carbohydrates: 1.7 g

· Fat: 1½ g

· Sugar: 0 g

Almond Flour Bread

Preparation Time: 10 minutes

2-Pound Loaf

Ingredients:

· 4 egg whites

· 2 egg yolks

· 2 cups almond flour

· ¼ cup butter, melted

· 2 tablespoons psyllium husk powder

· 1½ tablespoons baking powder

· ½ teaspoon Xanthan gum

· ¼ teaspoon salt

· ½ cup + 2 tablespoons warm water

· 2¼ teaspoons yeast

Directions:

1.Use a mixing bowl to combine all of the dry ingredients except for the yeast.

2.In the bread machine pan, add all the wet ingredients.

3.Add all of your dry ingredients from the small mixing bowl to the bread machine pan.

4.Set the machine to the basic setting.

5. When the bread is finished, remove it from the machine pan from the bread machine.

6.Let cool slightly before transferring to a cooling rack.

7.It can be stored for four days on the counter and three months in the freezer.

Nutrition:

· Calories: 215

· Sodium: 60 mg

· Carbohydrates: 2.4 g

· Protein: 4 g

Coconut Flour Bread

Preparation Time: 10 minutes

1½ -Pound Loaf

Ingredients:

· 6 eggs

· ½ cup coconut flour

· 2 tablespoons psyllium husk

· ¼ cup olive oil

· 1½ teaspoon salt

· 1 tablespoon Xanthan gum

· 1 tablespoon baking powder

· 2¼ teaspoons yeast

Directions:

1.Use a small bowl to combine all of the dry ingredients except for the yeast.

2.In the bread machine pan, add all the wet ingredients.

3.Add all of your dry ingredients from the small mixing bowl to the bread machine pan. Top with the yeast.

4.Set the machine to the basic setting.

5.When the bread is finished, remove the bread machine pan from the bread machine.

6.Let cool slightly before transferring to a cooling rack.

7.It can be stored for four days on the counter and up to 3 months in the freezer.

Nutrition:

· Calories: 214

· Sodium: 360 mg

· Carbohydrates: 4 g

· Protein: 7g

· Fat: 15 g

Flax Bread

Preparation Time: 45 minutes

1½-Pound Loaf

Ingredients:

· ¾ cup of water

· 10 g ground flax seeds

· ½ cup psyllium husk powder

· 1 tablespoon baking powder

· 7 large egg whites

· 3 tablespoons butter

· 2 teaspoons salt

· ¼ cup granulated stevia

· 1 large whole egg

· 1½ cups whey Protein: isolate

Directions:

1.Preheat the oven to 350⁰ F.

2.Combine whey Protein: isolate, psyllium husk, baking powder, sweetener, and salt.

3.In another bowl, mix the water, butter, egg, and egg whites.

4.Slowly add psyllium husk mixture to the egg mixture and mix well.

5. Grease the pan lightly with butter and pour in the batter.

6.Bake in the oven until the bread is set, about 1 to 1 ½ minute.

Nutrition:

· Calories: 265

· Sodium: 480 mg

· Fat: 15 g

· Carbohydrates: 5 g

· Protein: 24 g

Warm Spiced Pumpkin Bread

Preparation Time: 45 minutes

1½-Pound Loaf

Ingredients:

· 1½ cups pumpkin purée

· 3 eggs, at room temperature

· 1/3 cup melted butter cooled

· 1 cup of sugar

· 3 cups all-purpose flour

· 1½ teaspoons baking powder

· ¾ teaspoon ground cinnamon

· ½ teaspoon baking soda

· ¼ teaspoon ground nutmeg

· ¼ teaspoon ground ginger

· ¼ teaspoon salt

· Pinch ground cloves

Directions:

1.Lightly grease the bread bucket with butter.

2.Add the pumpkin, eggs, butter, and sugar.

3.Program the machine for Quick/Rapid setting and press Start.

4. Let the wet ingredients be mixed by the paddles until the first fast mixing cycle is finished, about 5 minutes into the process.

5.While the wet ingredients are mixing, stir together the flour, baking powder, cinnamon, baking soda, nutmeg, ginger, salt, and cloves until well blended.

6.Add the dry ingredients to the bucket when the second fast mixing cycle starts.

7.Scrape down the sides of the bucket once after the dry ingredients are mixed into the wet.

8.When the pound is finished, remove the bucket from the machine.

9.Let it cool for 5 minutes.

10.Gently shake the bucket to remove the bread and turn it out onto a rack to cool.

Nutrition:

· Calories: 251

·   Fat: 7g

· Carbohydrates: 43g

· Fiber: 2g

· Sodium: 159 mg

Multigrain Bread

Preparation Time: 15 minutes

1½-Pound Loaf

Ingredients:

· ¾ cups of water

· 1 tablespoon melted butter cooled

· ½ tablespoon honey

· ½ teaspoon salt

· ¾ cup multigrain flour

· 11/3 cups white bread flour

· 1 teaspoon bread machine or active dry yeast

Directions:

1.Place the ingredients in the device as recommended by the manufacturer.

2.Program the machine for a Basic White bread, select light or medium crust, then press the Start button.

3.When the pound is finished, remove the bucket from the machine.

4.Let it cool for five minutes.

5.Gently shake the bucket to remove the bread and turn it out onto a rack to cool.

Nutrition:

· Calories: 165

· Fat: 2 g

· Carbohydrates: 27 g

· Fiber: 1 g

· Sodium: 205 mg

· Protein: 4 g

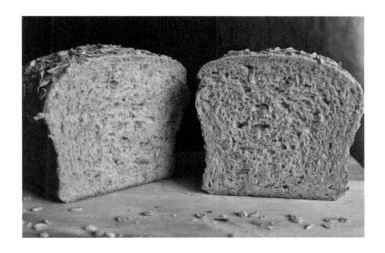